Jumping Jacks & Hula Hoops

Jumping Jacks & Hula Hoops

Karen Aken

ISBN-13: 978-1542857031
ISBN-10: 1542857031
Design by Mercedes Maynard

Introduction

Healthy is not skinny. Healthy is strong, energized, and happy. Jumping Jacks & Hula Hoops is not your typical book, it is a daily guide to better health for kids. This guide focuses on increasing physical activity; eating fruits and vegetables; staying well hydrated; setting goals; and keeping a positive attitude. Please consult your doctor before beginning this or any other healthy lifestyle program.

Day One

- Drink 6-8 glasses of water* (no flavor added, just WATER).
- Walk **or** jog (anywhere, inside or out) **or** march in place for at least 5 minutes.**
- Shut off all electronics for 2 minutes. Close your eyes. Inhale slowly and deeply to the count of 4, then exhale slowly to the count of 4 (breathe this way until time is up).**
- Think of something you are thankful for today.

*Never drink 6-8 glasses of water all at once, this can be harmful to your health. Please drink your water at a slow pace throughout the day.

**Ask a friend or family member to join you with these activities every day.

Day Two

- Drink 6-8 glasses of water (no flavor added, just WATER).
- Walk <u>or</u> jog (anywhere, inside or out) <u>or</u> march in place for at least 5 minutes.
- Shut off all electronics for 2 minutes. Close your eyes. Inhale slowly and deeply to the count of 4, then exhale slowly to the count of 4.
- Think of something you are thankful for today.
- **Stand on one leg and count to 10, stand on the other and count to 10.***

*This will improve your balance and also works your stomach muscles also known as your abs or core.

Day Three

- Drink 6-8 glasses of water (no flavor added, just WATER).
- Walk or jog (anywhere, inside or out) or march in place for at least 5 minutes.
- Shut off all electronics for 2 minutes. Close your eyes. Inhale slowly and deeply to the count of 4, then exhale slowly to the count of 4.
- Think of something you are thankful for today.
- Stand on one leg and count to 10, stand on the other and count to 10.
- **Do 10 Jumping Jacks.***

*This is a cardiovascular exercise also known as cardio. Cardiovascular exercise is any exercise that increases your heart rate.

Day Four

- Drink 6-8 glasses of water (no flavor added, just WATER).
- Walk <u>or</u> jog (anywhere, inside or out) <u>or</u> march in place for at least 5 minutes.
- Shut off all electronics for 2 minutes. Close your eyes. Inhale slowly and deeply to the count of 4, then exhale slowly to the count of 4.
- Think of something you are thankful for today.
- Stand on one leg and count to 10, stand on the other and count to 10.
- Do 10 Jumping Jacks.
- **Eat at least one whole piece of fruit (an apple, banana, orange, or whatever your favorite fruit is). Always wash fruits and vegetables before eating.**

*Health Tip: Never go more than 4 hours without eating (unless you are sleeping). After 4 hours your body slows down it's metabolism because it thinks it will starve. This also happens when you don't eat breakfast. A slow metabolism can make you gain weight.

Day Five

- Drink 6-8 glasses of water (no flavor added, just WATER).
- Walk <u>or</u> jog (anywhere, inside or out) <u>or</u> march in place for at least 5 minutes.
- Shut off all electronics for 2 minutes. Close your eyes. Inhale slowly and deeply to the count of 4, then exhale slowly to the count of 4.
- Think of something you are thankful for today.
- Stand on one leg and count to 10, stand on the other and count to 10.
- Do 10 Jumping Jacks.
- Eat at least one whole piece of fruit.
- **Do 5 sit-ups <u>or</u> hula hoop for 15 seconds in one direction and 15 seconds in the other direction (you don't have to have a hula hoop, you can pretend that you are using one).***

*These exercises improve your stomach muscles. They also improve your balance and help your body move better.
**Brain Challenge: Use your left hand when you eat dinner tonight (if you are right handed), if you are left handed use your right hand.

Day Six

- Drink 6-8 glasses of water (no flavor added, just WATER).
- Walk or jog (anywhere, inside or out) or march in place for at least 5 minutes.
- Shut off all electronics for 2 minutes. Close your eyes. Inhale slowly and deeply to the count of 4, then exhale slowly to the count of 4.
- Think of something you are thankful for today.
- Stand on one leg and count to 10, stand on the other and count to 10.
- Do 10 Jumping Jacks.
- Eat at least one whole piece of fruit.
- Do 5 sit-ups or hula hoop for 15 seconds in one direction and 15 seconds in the other direction.

*Health Tip: Let the grocery shopper in your home know that generic and store brands often contain more high fructose corn syrup (HFCS) than other brands. Eating or drinking products that contain HFCS is not good for your health.

Day Seven

- Drink 6-8 glasses of water (no flavor added, just WATER).
- Walk <u>or</u> jog (anywhere, inside or out) <u>or</u> march in place for at least 5 minutes.
- Shut off all electronics for 3 minutes. Close your eyes. Inhale slowly and deeply to the count of 4, then exhale slowly to the count of 4.
- Think of something you are thankful for today.
- Stand on one leg and count to 10, stand on the other and count to 10.
- Do 10 Jumping Jacks.
- Eat at least one whole piece of fruit.
- Do 5 sit-ups <u>or</u> hula hoop for 15 seconds in one direction and 15 seconds in the other direction.

*Have you wondered what this exercise is for? You have been practicing meditation. This is one of the best and easiest ways to improve the health of your mind and your body.

Day Eight

- Drink 6-8 glasses of water (no flavor added, just WATER).
- Walk or jog (anywhere, inside or out) or march in place for at least 5 minutes.
- Shut off all electronics for 3 minutes. Close your eyes. Inhale slowly and deeply to the count of 4, then exhale slowly to the count of 4.
- Think of something you are thankful for today.
- Stand on one leg and count to 10, stand on the other and count to 10.
- Do 10 Jumping Jacks.
- Eat at least one whole piece of fruit.
- Do 5 sit-ups or hula hoop for 15 seconds in one direction and 15 seconds in the other direction.
- Think of something you like about yourself.

*Health Tip: Singing burns calories (about 10 calories per song) and exercises your heart and your lungs. It can also cheer you up.

Day Nine

- Drink 6-8 glasses of water (no flavor added, just WATER).
- Walk _or_ jog (anywhere, inside or out) _or_ march in place for at least 5 minutes.
- Shut off all electronics for **3** minutes. Close your eyes. Inhale slowly and deeply to the count of 4, then exhale slowly to the count of 4.
- Think of something you are thankful for today.
- Stand on one leg and count to **15**, stand on the other and count to **15.**
- Do 10 Jumping Jacks.
- Eat at least one whole piece of fruit.
- Do 5 sit-ups _or_ hula hoop for 15 seconds in one direction and 15 seconds in the other direction.
- Think of something you like about yourself.

*Health Tip: Let the cook in your family know that ground turkey is healthier than ground beef. Ground turkey has less saturated fats. Saturated fats are not good for your heart or your body.

Day Ten

- Drink 6-8 glasses of water (no flavor added, just WATER).
- Walk or jog (anywhere, inside or out) or march in place for at least 5 minutes.
- Shut off all electronics for 3 minutes. Close your eyes. Inhale slowly and deeply to the count of 4, then exhale slowly to the count of 4.
- Think of something you are thankful for today.
- Stand on one leg and count to 15, stand on the other and count to 15.
- Do 10 Jumping Jacks.
- Eat at least one whole piece of fruit.
- Do 5 sit-ups or hula hoop for 15 seconds in one direction and 15 seconds in the other direction.
- Think of something you like about yourself.

*Health Tip: Gatorade and other sports drinks are just as unhealthy as soda. It is not a good idea to drink sports drinks unless you are playing a sport, running, or exercising for long periods of time (over 60 minutes) or spending a lot of time outside when it's hot.

Day Eleven

- Drink 6-8 glasses of water (no flavor added, just WATER).
- Go for a walk, jog or march in place for at least 7 minutes.
- Shut off all electronics for 3 minutes. Close your eyes. Inhale slowly and deeply to the count of 4, then exhale slowly to the count of 4.
- Think of something you are thankful for today.
- Stand on one leg and count to 15, stand on the other and count to 15.
- Do 10 Jumping Jacks.
- Eat at least one whole piece of fruit.
- Do 5 sit-ups <u>or</u> hula hoop for 15 seconds in one direction and 15 seconds in the other direction.
- Think of something you like about yourself.
- **Eat at least one 1/2 cup of vegetables (peas, green beans, carrots, or whatever your favorite vegetable is).**

*Health Tip: Let the cook in your family know that frozen fruits and vegetables are healthier than canned because they contain less salt and sugar. They also cost less.

Day Twelve

- Drink 6-8 glasses of water (no flavor added, just WATER).
- Go for a walk, jog or march in place for at least 7 minutes.
- Shut off all electronics for 3 minutes. Close your eyes. Inhale slowly and deeply to the count of 4, then exhale slowly to the count of 4.
- Think of something you are thankful for today.
- Stand on one leg and count to 15, stand on the other and count to 15.
- Do 10 Jumping Jacks.
- Eat at least one whole piece of fruit.
- Do **10** sit-ups or hula hoop for **20** seconds in one direction and **20** seconds in the other direction.
- Think of something you like about yourself.
- **Eat at least one 1/2 cup of vegetables.**

*Health Tip: Turning off all of your electronic devices at least 30 minutes before you go to bed and dimming the lights will help you fall asleep faster.

Day Thirteen

- Drink 6-8 glasses of water (no flavor added, just WATER).
- Go for a walk, jog or march in place for at least 7 minutes.
- Shut off all electronics for 3 minutes. Close your eyes. Inhale slowly and deeply to the count of 4, then exhale slowly to the count of 4.
- Think of something you are thankful for today.
- Stand on one leg and count to 15, stand on the other and count to 15.
- Do 10 Jumping Jacks.
- Eat at least one whole piece of fruit.
- Do 10 sit-ups <u>or</u> hula hoop for 20 seconds in one direction and 20 seconds in the other direction.
- Think of something you like about yourself.
- Eat at least one 1/2 cup of vegetables.

*Health Tip: Fat is not always bad for you. Your body needs fat for things like energy and to keep you warm. Vegetables, nuts, seeds, and fish contain healthy (good) fats. Cookies, cake, and chips contain unhealthy (bad) fats.

Day Fourteen

- Drink 6-8 glasses of water (no flavor added, just WATER).
- Go for a walk, jog or march in place for at least 7 minutes.
- Shut off all electronics for **4** minutes. Close your eyes. Inhale slowly and deeply to the count of 4, then exhale slowly to the count of 4.
- Think of something you are thankful for today.
- Stand on one leg and count to 15, stand on the other and count to 15.
- Do 10 Jumping Jacks.
- Eat at least one whole piece of fruit.
- Do 10 sit-ups or hula hoop for 20 seconds in one direction and 20 seconds in the other direction.
- Think of something you like about yourself.
- Eat at least one 1/2 cup of vegetables.
- **Do something nice for someone else.***

*Health Tip: The easiest way to feel good instantly is to do something nice for someone else.

Day Fifteen

- Drink 6-8 glasses of water (no flavor added, just WATER).
- Go for a walk, jog or march in place for at least **9** minutes.
- Shut off all electronics for 4 minutes. Close your eyes. Inhale slowly and deeply to the count of 4, then exhale slowly to the count of 4.
- Think of something you are thankful for today.
- Stand on one leg and count to **20**, stand on the other and count to **20**.
- Do 10 Jumping Jacks.
- Eat at least one whole piece of fruit.
- Do 10 sit-ups <u>or</u> hula hoop for 20 seconds in one direction and 20 seconds in the other direction.
- Think of something you like about yourself.
- Eat at least one 1/2 cup of vegetables.
- Do something nice for someone else.

*Brain challenge: Open cupboards, drawers, and doors without using your hands (at home).

Day Sixteen

- Drink 6-8 glasses of water (no flavor added, just WATER).
- Go for a walk, jog or march in place for at least 9 minutes.
- Shut off all electronics for 4 minutes. Close your eyes. Inhale slowly and deeply to the count of 4, then exhale slowly to the count of 4.
- Think of something you are thankful for today.
- Stand on one leg and count to 20, stand on the other and count to 20.
- Do 10 Jumping Jacks.
- Eat at least one whole piece of fruit.
- Do 10 sit-ups or hula hoop for 20 seconds in one direction and 20 seconds in the other direction.
- Think of something you like about yourself.
- Eat at least one 1/2 cup of vegetables.
- Do something nice for someone else.

*Just for today, every time you go to your room hop to get there.

Day Seventeen

- Drink 6-8 glasses of water (no flavor added, just WATER).
- Go for a walk, jog or march in place for at least 9 minutes.
- Shut off all electronics for 4 minutes. Close your eyes. Inhale slowly and deeply to the count of 4, then exhale slowly to the count of 4.
- Think of something you are thankful for today.
- Stand on one leg and count to 20, stand on the other and count to 20.
- Do **20** Jumping Jacks.
- Eat at least one whole piece of fruit.
- Do 10 sit-ups <u>or</u> hula hoop for 20 seconds in one direction and 20 seconds in the other direction.
- Think of something you like about yourself.
- Eat at least one 1/2 cup of vegetables.
- Do something nice for someone else.

*Health Tip: Red fruits and vegetables are good for your heart.

Day Eighteen

- Drink 6-8 glasses of water (no flavor added, just WATER).
- Go for a walk, jog or march in place for at least 9 minutes.
- Shut off all electronics for 4 minutes. Close your eyes. Inhale slowly and deeply to the count of 4, then exhale slowly to the count of 4.
- Think of something you are thankful for today.
- Stand on one leg and count to 20, stand on the other and count to 20.
- Do 20 Jumping Jacks.
- Eat **two** whole pieces of fruit.
- Do 10 sit-ups or hula hoop for 20 seconds in one direction and 20 seconds in the other direction.
- Think of something you like about yourself.
- Eat at least one 1/2 cup of vegetables.
- Do something nice for someone else.

*Health tip: Going to bed at the same time and waking up at the same time every day is a simple way to improve your health and improve your sleep.

Day Nineteen

- Drink 6-8 glasses of water (no flavor added, just WATER).
- Go for a walk, jog or march in place for at least 9 minutes.
- Shut off all electronics for 4 minutes. Close your eyes. Inhale slowly and deeply to the count of 4, then exhale slowly to the count of 4.
- Think of something you are thankful for today.
- Stand on one leg and count to 20, stand on the other and count to 20.
- Do 20 Jumping Jacks.
- Eat two whole pieces of fruit.
- Do **15** sit-ups <u>or</u> hula hoop for **25** seconds in one direction and **25** seconds in the other direction.
- Think of something you like about yourself.
- Eat at least one 1/2 cup of vegetables.
- Do something nice for someone else.

*Health Tip: Listening to music helps motivate you, improves your memory, and puts you in a good mood.

Day Twenty

- Drink 6-8 glasses of water (no flavor added, just WATER).
- Go for a walk, jog or march in place for at least 9 minutes.
- Shut off all electronics for 4 minutes. Close your eyes. Inhale slowly and deeply to the count of 4, then exhale slowly to the count of 4.
- Think of something you are thankful for today.
- Stand on one leg and count to 20, stand on the other and count to 20.
- Do 20 Jumping Jacks.
- Eat two whole pieces of fruit.
- Do 15 sit-ups or hula hoop for 25 seconds in one direction and 25 seconds in the other direction.
- Think of something you like about yourself.
- Eat at least one 1/2 cup of vegetables.
- Do something nice for someone else.

*Health Tip: Make a rule for yourself that if you are going to snack while you are online or watching TV, you will only snack on fruits or vegetables.

Day Twenty-One

- Drink 6-8 glasses of water (no flavor added, just WATER).
- Go for a walk, jog or march in place for at least 9 minutes.
- Shut off all electronics for 4 minutes. Close your eyes. Inhale slowly and deeply to the count of 4, then exhale slowly to the count of 4.
- Think of something you are thankful for today.
- Stand on one leg and count to 20, stand on the other and count to 20.
- Do 20 Jumping Jacks.
- Eat two whole pieces of fruit.
- Do 15 sit-ups or hula hoop for 25 seconds in one direction and 25 seconds in the other direction.
- Think of something you like about yourself.
- Eat at least one 1/2 cup of vegetables.
- Do something nice for someone else.
- **With your arms straight out from your sides, do arm circles 10 forward, 10 backward, big or small.**
- **Decide on a goal (example: quit drinking soda).**

*Just for today, every time you go to your kitchen, skip to get there.

Day Twenty-Two

- Drink 6-8 glasses of water (no flavor added, just WATER).
- Go for a walk, jog or march in place for at least **11** minutes.
- Shut off all electronics for 4 minutes. Close your eyes. Inhale slowly and deeply to the count of 4, then exhale slowly to the count of 4.
- Think of something you are thankful for today.
- Stand on one leg and count to 20, stand on the other and count to 20.
- Do 20 Jumping Jacks.
- Eat two whole pieces of fruit.
- Do 15 sit-ups or hula hoop for 25 seconds in one direction and 25 seconds in the other direction.
- Think of something you like about yourself.
- Eat at least one 1/2 cup of vegetables.
- Do something nice for someone else.
- With your arms straight out from your sides, do arm circles 10 forward, 10 backward, big or small.
- Work on achieving your goal.

*Health Tip: Swinging on a swing burns 50 calories in 15 minutes.

Day Twenty-Three

- Drink 6-8 glasses of water (no flavor added, just WATER).
- Go for a walk, jog or march in place for at least 11 minutes.
- Shut off all electronics for 4 minutes. Close your eyes. Inhale slowly and deeply to the count of 4, then exhale slowly to the count of 4.
- Think of something you are thankful for today.
- Stand on one leg and count to **25**, stand on the other and count to **25**.
- Do 20 Jumping Jacks.
- Eat two whole pieces of fruit.
- Do 15 sit-ups or hula hoop for 25 seconds in one direction and 25 seconds in the other direction.
- Think of something you like about yourself.
- Eat at least one 1/2 cup of vegetables.
- Do something nice for someone else.
- With your arms straight out from your sides, do arm circles 10 forward, 10 backward, big or small.
- Work on achieving your goal.

*Health Tip: Purple and blue fruits and vegetables are good for your heart, eyes, and skin.

Day Twenty-Four

- Drink 6-8 glasses of water (no flavor added, just WATER).
- Go for a walk, jog or march in place for at least 11 minutes.
- Shut off all electronics for 4 minutes. Close your eyes. Inhale slowly and deeply to the count of 4, then exhale slowly to the count of 4.
- Think of something you are thankful for today.
- Stand on one leg and count to 25, stand on the other and count to 25.*
- Do **25** Jumping Jacks.
- Eat two whole pieces of fruit.
- Do 15 sit-ups <u>or</u> hula hoop for 25 seconds in one direction and 25 seconds in the other direction.
- Think of something you like about yourself.
- Eat at least one 1/2 cup of vegetables.
- Do something nice for someone else.
- With your arms straight out from your sides, do arm circles 10 forward, 10 backward, big or small.
- Work on achieving your goal.

*Health Tip: To make standing on one leg more of a challenge, close your eyes.

Day Twenty-Five

- Drink 6-8 glasses of water (no flavor added, just WATER).
- Go for a walk, jog or march in place for at least 11 minutes.
- Shut off all electronics for 4 minutes. Close your eyes. Inhale slowly and deeply to the count of 4, then exhale slowly to the count of 4.
- Think of something you are thankful for today.
- Stand on one leg and count to 25, stand on the other and count to 25.
- Do 25 Jumping Jacks.
- Eat two whole pieces of fruit.
- Do 15 sit-ups <u>or</u> hula hoop for 25 seconds in one direction and 25 seconds in the other direction.
- Think of something you like about yourself.
- Eat at least **one** cup of vegetables.
- Do something nice for someone else.
- With your arms straight out from your sides, do arm circles 10 forward, 10 backward, big or small.
- Work on achieving your goal.

*Brain Challenge: Say your ABC's backwards.

Day Twenty-Six

- Drink 6-8 glasses of water (no flavor added, just WATER).
- Go for a walk, jog or march in place for at least 11 minutes.
- Shut off all electronics for 4 minutes. Close your eyes. Inhale slowly and deeply to the count of 4, then exhale slowly to the count of 4.
- Think of something you are thankful for today.
- Stand on one leg and count to 25, stand on the other and count to 25.
- Do 25 Jumping Jacks.
- Eat two whole pieces of fruit.
- Do **20** sit-ups <u>or</u> hula hoop for **30** seconds in one direction and **30** seconds in the other direction.
- Think of something you like about yourself.
- Eat at least one cup of vegetables.
- Do something nice for someone else.
- With your arms straight out from your sides, do arm circles 10 forward, 10 backward, big or small.
- Work on achieving your goal.

*Health Tip: Eat breakfast within 2 hours of waking up to give your body and your brain energy. The sooner the better!

Day Twenty-Seven

- Drink 6-8 glasses of water (no flavor added, just WATER).
- Go for a walk, jog or march in place for at least 11 minutes.
- Shut off all electronics for 4 minutes. Close your eyes. Inhale slowly and deeply to the count of 4, then exhale slowly to the count of 4.
- Think of something you are thankful for today.
- Stand on one leg and count to 25, stand on the other and count to 25.
- Do 25 Jumping Jacks.
- Eat two whole pieces of fruit.
- Do 20 sit-ups or hula hoop for 30 seconds in one direction and 30 seconds in the other direction.
- Think of something you like about yourself.
- Eat at least one cup of vegetables.
- Do something nice for someone else.
- With your arms straight out from your sides, do arm circles 10 forward, 10 backward, big or small.
- Work on achieving your goal.

*Health Tip: Orange fruits and vegetables are good for your eyes and your skin. They also strengthen your immunity (help you avoid getting sick).

Day Twenty-Eight

- Drink 6-8 glasses of water (no flavor added, just WATER).
- Go for a walk, jog or march in place for at least 11 minutes.
- Shut off all electronics for **6** minutes. Close your eyes. Inhale slowly and deeply to the count of 4, then exhale slowly to the count of 4.
- Think of something you are thankful for today.
- Stand on one leg and count to 25, stand on the other and count to 25.
- Do 25 Jumping Jacks.
- Eat two whole pieces of fruit.
- Do 20 sit-ups or hula hoop for 30 seconds in one direction and 30 seconds in the other direction.
- Think of something you like about yourself.
- Eat at least one cup of vegetables.
- Do something nice for someone else.
- With your arms straight out from your sides, do arm circles **15** forward, **15** backward, big **and** small.
- Work on achieving your goal.

*Health Tip: Staying well hydrated prevents headaches.

Day Twenty-Nine

- Drink 6-8 glasses of water (no flavor added, just WATER).
- Go for a walk, jog or march in place for at least **13** minutes.
- Shut off all electronics for 6 minutes. Close your eyes. Inhale slowly and deeply to the count of 4, then exhale slowly to the count of 4.
- Think of something you are thankful for today.
- Stand on one leg and count to 25, stand on the other and count to 25.
- Do 25 Jumping Jacks.
- Eat two whole pieces of fruit.
- Do 20 sit-ups <u>or</u> hula hoop for 30 seconds in one direction and 30 seconds in the other direction.
- Think of something you like about yourself.
- Eat at least one cup of vegetables.
- Do something nice for someone else.
- With your arms straight out from your sides, do arm circles 15 forward, 15 backward, big and small.
- Work on achieving your goal.

*Avoid all electronics today (except for any electronics you need to use for school).

Day Thirty

- Drink 6-8 glasses of water (no flavor added, just WATER).
- Go for a walk, jog or march in place for at least 13 minutes.
- Shut off all electronics for 6 minutes. Close your eyes. Inhale slowly and deeply to the count of 4, then exhale slowly to the count of 4.
- Think of something you are thankful for today.
- Stand on one leg and count to **30**, stand on the other and count to **30**.
- Do 25 Jumping Jacks.
- Eat two whole pieces of fruit.
- Do 20 sit-ups or hula hoop for 30 seconds in one direction and 30 seconds in the other direction.
- Think of something you like about yourself.
- Eat at least one cup of vegetables.
- Do something nice for someone else.
- With your arms straight out from your sides, do arm circles 15 forward, 15 backward, big and small.
- Work on achieving your goal.

*Health Tip: Smile! It makes you happy and relaxes your body.

Day Thirty-One

- Drink 6-8 glasses of water (no flavor added, just WATER).
- Go for a walk, jog or march in place for at least 13 minutes.
- Shut off all electronics for 6 minutes. Close your eyes. Inhale slowly and deeply to the count of 4, then exhale slowly to the count of 4.
- Think of something you are thankful for today.
- Stand on one leg and count to 30, stand on the other and count to 30.
- Do **30** Jumping Jacks.
- Eat two whole pieces of fruit.
- Do 20 sit-ups <u>or</u> hula hoop for 30 seconds in one direction and 30 seconds in the other direction.
- Think of something you like about yourself.
- Eat at least one cup of vegetables.
- Do something nice for someone else.
- With your arms straight out from your sides, do arm circles 15 forward, 15 backward, big and small.
- Work on achieving your goal.

*Health Tip: White fruits and vegetables are good for your bones.

Day Thirty-Two

- Drink 6-8 glasses of water (no flavor added, just WATER).
- Go for a walk, jog or march in place for at least 13 minutes.
- Shut off all electronics for 6 minutes. Close your eyes. Inhale slowly and deeply to the count of 4, then exhale slowly to the count of 4.
- Think of something you are thankful for today.
- Stand on one leg and count to 30, stand on the other and count to 30.
- Do 30 Jumping Jacks.
- Eat two whole pieces of fruit.
- Do 20 sit-ups or hula hoop for 30 seconds in one direction and 30 seconds in the other direction.
- Think of something you like about yourself.
- Eat at least **one and a 1/2 cups** of vegetables.
- Do something nice for someone else.
- With your arms straight out from your sides, do arm circles 15 forward, 15 backward, big and small.
- Work on achieving your goal.

*Just for today, every time you sit down (while you are at home), stand up and sit down again 3x.

Day Thirty-Three

- Drink 6-8 glasses of water (no flavor added, just WATER).
- Go for a walk, jog or march in place for at least 13 minutes.
- Shut off all electronics for 6 minutes. Close your eyes. Inhale slowly and deeply to the count of 4, then exhale slowly to the count of 4.
- Think of something you are thankful for today.
- Stand on one leg and count to 30, stand on the other and count to 30.
- Do 30 Jumping Jacks.
- Eat two whole pieces of fruit.
- Do **25** sit-ups <u>or</u> hula hoop for **35** seconds in one direction and **35** seconds in the other direction.
- Think of something you like about yourself.
- Eat at least one and a 1/2 cups of vegetables.
- Do something nice for someone else.
- With your arms straight out from your sides, do arm circles 15 forward, 15 backward, big and small.
- Work on achieving your goal.

*Health Tip: Try balancing on one leg and then the other while brushing your teeth.

Day Thirty-Four

- Drink 6-8 glasses of water (no flavor added, just WATER).
- Go for a walk, jog or march in place for at least 13 minutes.
- Shut off all electronics for 6 minutes. Close your eyes. Inhale slowly and deeply to the count of 4, then exhale slowly to the count of 4.
- Think of something you are thankful for today.
- Stand on one leg and count to 30, stand on the other and count to 30.
- Do 30 Jumping Jacks.
- Eat two whole pieces of fruit.
- Do 25 sit-ups or hula hoop for 35 seconds in one direction and 35 seconds in the other direction.
- Think of something you like about yourself.
- Eat at least one and a 1/2 cups of vegetables.
- Do something nice for someone else.
- With your arms straight out from your sides, do arm circles 15 forward, 15 backward, big and small.
- Work on achieving your goal.

*Health Tip: Even your eyes can be at risk for sunburn. Wearing sunglasses can prevent eye problems now and later on in life.

Day Thirty-Five

- Drink 6-8 glasses of water (no flavor added, just WATER).
- Go for a walk, jog or march in place for at least 13 minutes.
- Shut off all electronics for 6 minutes. Close your eyes. Inhale slowly and deeply to the count of 4, then exhale slowly to the count of 4.
- Think of something you are thankful for today.
- Stand on one leg and count to 30, stand on the other and count to 30.
- Do 30 Jumping Jacks.
- Eat two whole pieces of fruit.
- Do 25 sit-ups or hula hoop for 35 seconds in one direction and 35 seconds in the other direction.
- Think of something you like about yourself.
- Eat at least one and a 1/2 cups of vegetables.
- Do something nice for someone else.
- With your arms straight out from your sides, do arm circles 15 forward, 15 backward, big and small.
- Work on achieving your goal.
- **Time for another goal. If you have completed your first goal by now, it is okay to have two goals.**

*Brain Challenge: Brush your teeth with your left hand (if you are right handed), if you are left handed - use your right hand.

Day Thirty-Six

- Drink 6-8 glasses of water (no flavor added, just WATER).
- Go for a walk, jog or march in place for at least **15** minutes.
- Shut off all electronics for 6 minutes. Close your eyes. Inhale slowly and deeply to the count of 4, then exhale slowly to the count of 4.
- Think of something you are thankful for today.
- Stand on one leg and count to 30, stand on the other and count to 30.
- Do 30 Jumping Jacks.
- Eat two whole pieces of fruit.
- Do 25 sit-ups <u>or</u> hula hoop for 35 seconds in one direction and 35 seconds in the other direction.
- Think of something you like about yourself.
- Eat at least one and a 1/2 cups of vegetables.
- Do something nice for someone else.
- With your arms straight out from your sides, do arm circles **20** forward, **20** backward, big and small.
- Work on achieving your goal(s).

*Health Tip: Try standing on your tippy toes while brushing your teeth to improve balance.

Day Thirty-Seven

- Drink 6-8 glasses of water (no flavor added, just WATER).
- Go for a walk, jog or march in place for at least 15 minutes.
- Shut off all electronics for 6 minutes. Close your eyes. Inhale slowly and deeply to the count of 4, then exhale slowly to the count of 4.
- Think of something you are thankful for today.
- Stand on one leg and count to 30, stand on the other and count to 30.
- Do 30 Jumping Jacks.
- Eat two whole pieces of fruit.
- Do 25 sit-ups <u>or</u> hula hoop for 35 seconds in one direction and 35 seconds in the other direction.
- Think of something you like about yourself.
- Eat at least one and a 1/2 cups of vegetables.
- Do something nice for someone else.
- With your arms straight out from your sides, do arm circles 20 forward, 20 backward, big and small.
- Work on achieving your goal(s).
- **Hop** on one leg and count to **10**, then the other and count to **10.**

*Health Tip: Carbohydrates are good for you. Make sure you choose healthy carbs like whole grain bread, potatoes, fruits, and vegetables.

Day Thirty-Eight

- Drink 6-8 glasses of water (no flavor added, just WATER).
- Go for a walk, jog or march in place for at least 15 minutes.
- Shut off all electronics for 6 minutes. Close your eyes. Inhale slowly and deeply to the count of 4, then exhale slowly to the count of 4.
- Think of something you are thankful for today.
- Stand on one leg and count to 30, stand on the other and count to 30.
- Do **35** Jumping Jacks.
- Eat two whole pieces of fruit.
- Do 25 sit-ups <u>or</u> hula hoop for 35 seconds in one direction and 35 seconds in the other direction.
- Think of something you like about yourself.
- Eat at least one and a 1/2 cups of vegetables.
- Do something nice for someone else.
- With your arms straight out from your sides, do arm circles 20 forward, 20 backward, big and small.
- Work on achieving your goal(s).
- Hop on one leg and count to 10, then the other and count to 10.

*Just 5-15 minutes of sunlight on your hands, arms, and face 2 - 3x each week can make you happier, and strengthen your bones.

Day Thirty-Nine

- Drink 6-8 glasses of water (no flavor added, just WATER).
- Go for a walk, jog or march in place for at least 15 minutes.
- Shut off all electronics for 6 minutes. Close your eyes. Inhale slowly and deeply to the count of 4, then exhale slowly to the count of 4.
- Think of something you are thankful for today.
- Stand on one leg and count to 30, stand on the other and count to 30.
- Do 35 Jumping Jacks.
- Eat two whole pieces of fruit.
- Do 25 sit-ups or hula hoop for 35 seconds in one direction and 35 seconds in the other direction.
- Think of something you like about yourself.
- Eat at least one and a 1/2 cups of vegetables.
- Do something nice for someone else.
- With your arms straight out from your sides, do arm circles 20 forward, 20 backward, big and small.
- Work on achieving your goal(s).
- Hop on one leg and count to 10, then the other and count to 10.

*If you can't sleep at night because you think about your day or things that bother you, try keeping a notebook by your bed and write down those thoughts. This will help get those thoughts out of your head so you can sleep.

Day Forty

- Drink 6-8 glasses of water (no flavor added, just WATER).
- Go for a walk, jog or march in place for at least 15 minutes.
- Shut off all electronics for 6 minutes. Close your eyes. Inhale slowly and deeply to the count of 4, then exhale slowly to the count of 4.
- Think of something you are thankful for today.
- Stand on one leg and count to 30, stand on the other and count to 30.
- Do 35 Jumping Jacks.
- Eat two whole pieces of fruit.
- Do **30** sit-ups or hula hoop for **40** seconds in one direction and **40** seconds in the other direction.
- Think of something you like about yourself.
- Eat at least one and a 1/2 cups of vegetables.
- Do something nice for someone else.
- With your arms straight out from your sides, do arm circles 20 forward, 20 backward, big and small.
- Work on achieving your goal(s).
- Hop on one leg and count to 10, then the other and count to 10.

*Health Tip: Fiber helps your body digest food. It is found in fruits, vegetables, and whole grains.

Day Forty-One

- Drink 6-8 glasses of water (no flavor added, just WATER).
- Go for a walk, jog or march in place for at least 15 minutes.
- Shut off all electronics for 6 minutes. Close your eyes. Inhale slowly and deeply to the count of 4, then exhale slowly to the count of 4.
- Think of something you are thankful for today.
- Stand on one leg and count to 30, stand on the other and count to 30.
- Do 35 Jumping Jacks.
- Eat two whole pieces of fruit.
- Do 30 sit-ups or hula hoop for 40 seconds in one direction and 40 seconds in the other direction.
- Think of something you like about yourself.
- Eat at least one and a 1/2 cups of vegetables.
- Do something nice for someone else.
- With your arms straight out from your sides, do arm circles 20 forward, 20 backward, big and small.
- Work on achieving your goal(s).
- Hop on one leg and count to 10, then the other and count to 10.

*Just for today, every time you go to your room hop to get there.

Day Forty-Two

- Drink 6-8 glasses of water (no flavor added, just WATER).
- Go for a walk, jog or march in place for at least 15 minutes.
- Shut off all electronics for 6 minutes. Close your eyes. Inhale slowly and deeply to the count of 4, then exhale slowly to the count of 4.
- Think of something you are thankful for today.
- Stand on one leg and count to 30, stand on the other and count to 30.
- Do 35 Jumping Jacks.
- Eat two whole pieces of fruit.
- Do 30 sit-ups or hula hoop for 40 seconds in one direction and 40 seconds in the other direction.
- Think of something you like about yourself.
- Eat at least one and a 1/2 cups of vegetables.
- Do something nice for someone else.
- With your arms straight out from your sides, do arm circles **25** forward, **25** backward, big and small.
- Work on achieving your goal(s).
- Hop on one leg and count to 10, then the other and count to 10.

*Health Tip: When you are upset, inhale deeply for 5 seconds, hold it in for 3 seconds, and then exhale for 5 seconds. Repeat as necessary. This is one of the quickest and easiest ways to calm down.

Day Forty-Three

- Drink 6-8 glasses of water (no flavor added, just WATER).
- Go for a walk, jog or march in place for at least **17** minutes.
- Shut off all electronics for 6 minutes. Close your eyes. Inhale slowly and deeply to the count of 4, then exhale slowly to the count of 4.
- Think of something you are thankful for today.
- Stand on one leg and count to 30, stand on the other and count to 30.
- Do 35 Jumping Jacks.
- Eat two whole pieces of fruit.
- Do 30 sit-ups <u>or</u> hula hoop for 40 seconds in one direction and 40 seconds in the other direction.
- Think of something you like about yourself.
- Eat at least one and a 1/2 cups of vegetables.
- Do something nice for someone else.
- With your arms straight out from your sides, do arm circles 25 forward, 25 backward, big and small.
- Work on achieving your goal(s).
- Hop on one leg and count to 10, then the other and count to 10.

*Health Tip: Vitamins help your body stay healthy and fight disease. Vitamins are found in fruits, nuts and vegetables.

Day Forty-Four

- Drink 6-8 glasses of water (no flavor added, just WATER).
- Go for a walk, jog or march in place for at least 17 minutes.
- Shut off all electronics for 6 minutes. Close your eyes. Inhale slowly and deeply to the count of 4, then exhale slowly to the count of 4.
- Think of something you are thankful for today.
- Stand on one leg and count to 30, stand on the other and count to 30.
- Do 35 Jumping Jacks.
- Eat two whole pieces of fruit.
- Do 30 sit-ups or hula hoop for 40 seconds in one direction and 40 seconds in the other direction.
- Think of something you like about yourself.
- Eat at least one and a 1/2 cups of vegetables.
- Do something nice for someone else.
- With your arms straight out from your sides, do arm circles 25 forward, 25 backward, big and small.
- Work on achieving your goal(s).
- Hop on one leg and count to **15**, then the other and count to **15**.

*Health Tip: Carrots are good for your eyes and help to prevent you from getting sick.

Day Forty-Five

- Drink 6-8 glasses of water (no flavor added, just WATER).
- Go for a walk, jog or march in place for at least 17 minutes.
- Shut off all electronics for 6 minutes. Close your eyes. Inhale slowly and deeply to the count of 4, then exhale slowly to the count of 4.
- Think of something you are thankful for today.
- Stand on one leg and count to 30, stand on the other and count to 30.
- Do **40** Jumping Jacks.
- Eat two whole pieces of fruit.
- Do 30 sit-ups <u>or</u> hula hoop for 40 seconds in one direction and 40 seconds in the other direction.
- Think of something you like about yourself.
- Eat at least one and a 1/2 cups of vegetables.
- Do something nice for someone else.
- With your arms straight out from your sides, do arm circles 25 forward, 25 backward, big and small.
- Work on achieving your goal(s).
- Hop on one leg and count to 15, then the other and count to 15.

*Brain Challenge: Use your left hand when you eat dinner tonight (if you are right handed), if you are left handed use your right hand.

Day Forty-Six

- Drink 6-8 glasses of water (no flavor added, just WATER).
- Go for a walk, jog or march in place for at least 17 minutes.
- Shut off all electronics for 6 minutes. Close your eyes. Inhale slowly and deeply to the count of 4, then exhale slowly to the count of 4.
- Think of something you are thankful for today.
- Stand on one leg and count to 30, stand on the other and count to 30.
- Do 40 Jumping Jacks.
- Eat two whole pieces of fruit.
- Do 30 sit-ups or hula hoop for 40 seconds in one direction and 40 seconds in the other direction.
- Think of something you like about yourself.
- Eat at least one and a 1/2 cups of vegetables.
- Do something nice for someone else.
- With your arms straight out from your sides, do arm circles 25 forward, 25 backward, big and small.
- Work on achieving your goal(s).
- Hop on one leg and count to 15, then the other and count to 15.

*Health Tip: Bananas are good for your heart and can help improve your mood.

Day Forty-Seven

- Drink 6-8 glasses of water (no flavor added, just WATER).
- Go for a walk, jog or march in place for at least 17 minutes.
- Shut off all electronics for 6 minutes. Close your eyes. Inhale slowly and deeply to the count of 4, then exhale slowly to the count of 4.
- Think of something you are thankful for today.
- Stand on one leg and count to 30, stand on the other and count to 30.
- Do 40 Jumping Jacks.
- Eat two whole pieces of fruit.
- Do **35** sit-ups or hula hoop for **45** seconds in one direction and **45** seconds in the other direction.
- Think of something you like about yourself.
- Eat at least one and a 1/2 cups of vegetables.
- Do something nice for someone else.
- With your arms straight out from your sides, do arm circles 25 forward, 25 backward, big and small.
- Work on achieving your goal(s).
- Hop on one leg and count to 15, then the other and count to 15.

*Health Tip: Take your time eating. It takes 20 minutes for the message that you are full to get from your stomach to your brain.

Day Forty-Eight

- Drink 6-8 glasses of water (no flavor added, just WATER).
- Go for a walk, jog or march in place for at least 17 minutes.
- Shut off all electronics for 6 minutes. Close your eyes. Inhale slowly and deeply to the count of 4, then exhale slowly to the count of 4.
- Think of something you are thankful for today.
- Stand on one leg and count to 30, stand on the other and count to 30.
- Do 40 Jumping Jacks.
- Eat two whole pieces of fruit.
- Do 35 sit-ups or hula hoop for 45 seconds in one direction and 45 seconds in the other direction.
- Think of something you like about yourself.
- Eat at least one and a 1/2 cups of vegetables.
- Do something nice for someone else.
- With your arms straight out from your sides, do arm circles 25 forward, 25 backward, big and small.
- Work on achieving your goal(s).
- Hop on one leg and count to 15, then the other and count to 15.

*Health Tip: The more colors of foods you eat (fruits and vegetables - think red apple or green beans, etc.) the better your diet. Every fruit and vegetable offers different nutrients that help your body in different ways.

Day Forty-Nine

- Drink 6-8 glasses of water (no flavor added, just WATER).
- Go for a walk, jog or march in place for at least 17 minutes.
- Shut off all electronics for 6 minutes. Close your eyes. Inhale slowly and deeply to the count of 4, then exhale slowly to the count of 4.
- Think of something you are thankful for today.
- Stand on one leg and count to 30, stand on the other and count to 30.
- Do 40 Jumping Jacks.
- Eat two whole pieces of fruit.
- Do 35 sit-ups <u>or</u> hula hoop for 45 seconds in one direction and 45 seconds in the other direction.
- Think of something you like about yourself.
- Eat at least one and a 1/2 cups of vegetables.
- Do something nice for someone else.
- With your arms straight out from your sides, do arm circles **30** forward, **30** backward, big and small.
- Work on achieving your goal(s).
- Hop on one leg and count to 15, then the other and count to 15.

*Health Tip: Eat only when you are hungry, not when you are bored.

Day Fifty

- Drink 6-8 glasses of water (no flavor added, just WATER).
- Go for a walk, jog or march in place for at least **19** minutes.
- Shut off all electronics for 6 minutes. Close your eyes. Inhale slowly and deeply to the count of 4, then exhale slowly to the count of 4.
- Think of something you are thankful for today.
- Stand on one leg and count to 30, stand on the other and count to 30.
- Do 40 Jumping Jacks.
- Eat two whole pieces of fruit.
- Do 35 sit-ups or hula hoop for 45 seconds in one direction and 45 seconds in the other direction.
- Think of something you like about yourself.
- Eat at least one and a 1/2 cups of vegetables.
- Do something nice for someone else.
- With your arms straight out from your sides, do arm circles 30 forward, 30 backward, big and small.
- Work on achieving your goal(s).
- Hop on one leg and count to 15, then the other and count to 15.

*Just for today, every time you go to your kitchen, skip to get there.

Day Fifty-One

- Drink 6-8 glasses of water (no flavor added, just WATER).
- Go for a walk, jog or march in place for at least 19 minutes.
- Shut off all electronics for 6 minutes. Close your eyes. Inhale slowly and deeply to the count of 4, then exhale slowly to the count of 4.
- Think of something you are thankful for today.
- Stand on one leg and count to 30, stand on the other and count to 30.
- Do 40 Jumping Jacks.
- Eat two whole pieces of fruit.
- Do 35 sit-ups or hula hoop for 45 seconds in one direction and 45 seconds in the other direction.
- Think of something you like about yourself.
- Eat at least one and a 1/2 cups of vegetables.
- Do something nice for someone else.
- With your arms straight out from your sides, do arm circles 30 forward, 30 backward, big and small.
- Work on achieving your goal(s).
- Hop on one leg and count to **20**, then the other and count to **20**.

*Test Yourself: How many sit-ups can you do in 2 minutes?

Day Fifty-Two

- Drink 6-8 glasses of water (no flavor added, just WATER).
- Go for a walk, jog or march in place for at least 19 minutes.
- Shut off all electronics for 6 minutes. Close your eyes. Inhale slowly and deeply to the count of 4, then exhale slowly to the count of 4.
- Think of something you are thankful for today.
- Stand on one leg and count to 30, stand on the other and count to 30.
- Do **45** Jumping Jacks.
- Eat two whole pieces of fruit.
- Do 35 sit-ups <u>or</u> hula hoop for 45 seconds in one direction and 45 seconds in the other direction.
- Think of something you like about yourself.
- Eat at least one and a 1/2 cups of vegetables.
- Do something nice for someone else.
- With your arms straight out from your sides, do arm circles 30 forward, 30 backward, big and small.
- Work on achieving your goal(s).
- Hop on one leg and count to 20, then the other and count to 20.

*Test Yourself: How many jumping jacks can you do in 2 minutes?

Day Fifty-Three

- Drink 6-8 glasses of water (no flavor added, just WATER).
- Go for a walk, jog or march in place for at least 19 minutes.
- Shut off all electronics for 6 minutes. Close your eyes. Inhale slowly and deeply to the count of 4, then exhale slowly to the count of 4.
- Think of something you are thankful for today.
- Stand on one leg and count to 30, stand on the other and count to 30.
- Do 45 Jumping Jacks.
- Eat two whole pieces of fruit.
- Do 35 sit-ups or hula hoop for 45 seconds in one direction and 45 seconds in the other direction.
- Think of something you like about yourself.
- Eat at least one and a 1/2 cups of vegetables.
- Do something nice for someone else.
- With your arms straight out from your sides, do arm circles 30 forward, 30 backward, big and small.
- Work on achieving your goal(s).
- Hop on one leg and count to 20, then the other and count to 20.

*Test Yourself: How many push-ups can you do in 30 seconds?

Day Fifty-Four

- Drink 6-8 glasses of water (no flavor added, just WATER).
- Go for a walk, jog or march in place for at least 19 minutes.
- Shut off all electronics for 6 minutes. Close your eyes. Inhale slowly and deeply to the count of 4, then exhale slowly to the count of 4.
- Think of something you are thankful for today.
- Stand on one leg and count to 30, stand on the other and count to 30.
- Do 45 Jumping Jacks.
- Eat two whole pieces of fruit.
- Do **40** sit-ups <u>or</u> hula hoop for **50** seconds in one direction and **50** seconds in the other direction.
- Think of something you like about yourself.
- Eat at least one and a 1/2 cups of vegetables.
- Do something nice for someone else.
- With your arms straight out from your sides, do arm circles 30 forward, 30 backward, big and small.*
- Work on achieving your goal(s).
- Hop on one leg and count to 20, then the other and count to 20.

*To make arm circles more of a challenge, close your eyes and stand on one leg.

Day Fifty-Five

- Drink 6-8 glasses of water (no flavor added, just WATER).
- Go for a walk, jog or march in place for at least 19 minutes.
- Shut off all electronics for 6 minutes. Close your eyes. Inhale slowly and deeply to the count of 4, then exhale slowly to the count of 4.
- Think of something you are thankful for today.
- Stand on one leg and count to 30, stand on the other and count to 30.
- Do 45 Jumping Jacks.
- Eat two whole pieces of fruit.
- Do 40 sit-ups or hula hoop for 50 seconds in one direction and 50 seconds in the other direction.
- Think of something you like about yourself.
- Eat at least one and a 1/2 cups of vegetables.
- Do something nice for someone else.
- With your arms straight out from your sides, do arm circles 30 forward, 30 backward, big and small.
- Work on achieving your goal(s).
- Hop on one leg and count to 20, then the other and count to 20.

*Brain Challenge: Open cupboards, drawers, and doors without using your hands (at home).

Day Fifty-Six

- Drink 6-8 glasses of water (no flavor added, just WATER).
- Go for a walk, jog or march in place for at least 19 minutes.
- Shut off all electronics for 6 minutes. Close your eyes. Inhale slowly and deeply to the count of 4, then exhale slowly to the count of 4.
- Think of something you are thankful for today.
- Stand on one leg and count to 30, stand on the other and count to 30.
- Do 45 Jumping Jacks.
- Eat two whole pieces of fruit.
- Do 40 sit-ups or hula hoop for 50 seconds in one direction and 50 seconds in the other direction.
- Think of something you like about yourself.
- Eat at least one and a 1/2 cups of vegetables.
- Do something nice for someone else.
- With your arms straight out from your sides, do arm circles **20** forward, **20** backward, big and small.
- Work on achieving your goal(s).
- Hop on one leg and count to 20, then the other and count to 20.

*Health Tip: Protein helps build muscle and repair damage.

Day Fifty-Seven

- Drink 6-8 glasses of water (no flavor added, just WATER).
- Go for a walk, jog or march in place for at least **21** minutes.
- Shut off all electronics for 6 minutes. Close your eyes. Inhale slowly and deeply to the count of 4, then exhale slowly to the count of 4.
- Think of something you are thankful for today.
- Stand on one leg and count to 30, stand on the other and count to 30.
- Do 45 Jumping Jacks.
- Eat two whole pieces of fruit.
- Do 40 sit-ups or hula hoop for 50 seconds in one direction and 50 seconds in the other direction.
- Think of something you like about yourself.
- Eat at least one and a 1/2 cups of vegetables.
- Do something nice for someone else.
- With your arms straight out from your sides, do arm circles 20 forward, 20 backward, big and small.
- Work on achieving your goal(s).
- Hop on one leg and count to 20, then the other and count to 20.

*Health Tip: Laughing is good for your mind, body, and heart.

Day Fifty-Eight

- Drink 6-8 glasses of water (no flavor added, just WATER).
- Go for a walk, jog or march in place for at least 21 minutes.
- Shut off all electronics for 6 minutes. Close your eyes. Inhale slowly and deeply to the count of 4, then exhale slowly to the count of 4.
- Think of something you are thankful for today.
- Stand on one leg and count to 30, stand on the other and count to 30.
- Do 45 Jumping Jacks.
- Eat two whole pieces of fruit.
- Do 40 sit-ups or hula hoop for 50 seconds in one direction and 50 seconds in the other direction.
- Think of something you like about yourself.
- Eat at least one and a 1/2 cups of vegetables.
- Do something nice for someone else.
- With your arms straight out from your sides, do arm circles 20 forward, 20 backward, big and small.
- Work on achieving your goal(s).
- Hop on one leg and count to **25**, then the other and count to **25**.

*Health Tip: Jumping rope improves coordination, helps keep your bones strong, and burns more calories than jogging.

Day Fifty-Nine

- Drink 6-8 glasses of water (no flavor added, just WATER).
- Go for a walk, jog or march in place for at least 21 minutes.
- Shut off all electronics for 6 minutes. Close your eyes. Inhale slowly and deeply to the count of 4, then exhale slowly to the count of 4.
- Think of something you are thankful for today.
- Stand on one leg and count to 30, stand on the other and count to 30.
- Do **50** Jumping Jacks.
- Eat two whole pieces of fruit.
- Do 40 sit-ups <u>or</u> hula hoop for 50 seconds in one direction and 50 seconds in the other direction.
- Think of something you like about yourself.
- Eat at least one and a 1/2 cups of vegetables.
- Do something nice for someone else.
- With your arms straight out from your sides, do arm circles 20 forward, 20 backward, big and small.
- Work on achieving your goal(s).
- Hop on one leg and count to 25, then the other and count to 25.

*Just for today, every time you sit down (while you are at home), stand up and sit down again 3x.

Day Sixty

- Drink 6-8 glasses of water (no flavor added, just WATER).
- Go for a walk, jog or march in place for at least 21 minutes.
- Shut off all electronics for 6 minutes. Close your eyes. Inhale slowly and deeply to the count of 4, then exhale slowly to the count of 4.
- Think of something you are thankful for today.
- Stand on one leg and count to 30, stand on the other and count to 30.
- Do 50 Jumping Jacks.
- Eat two whole pieces of fruit.
- Do 40 sit-ups or hula hoop for 50 seconds in one direction and 50 seconds in the other direction.
- Think of something you like about yourself.
- Eat at least one and a 1/2 cups of vegetables.
- Do something nice for someone else.
- With your arms straight out from your sides, do arm circles 20 forward, 20 backward, big and small.
- Work on achieving your goal(s).
- Hop on one leg and count to 25, then the other and count to 25.

*Health Tip: Forgiving others is good for your heart.

Day Sixty-One

- Drink 6-8 glasses of water (no flavor added, just WATER).
- Go for a walk, jog or march in place for at least 21 minutes.
- Shut off all electronics for 6 minutes. Close your eyes. Inhale slowly and deeply to the count of 4, then exhale slowly to the count of 4.
- Think of something you are thankful for today.
- Stand on one leg and count to 30, stand on the other and count to 30.
- Do 50 Jumping Jacks.
- Eat two whole pieces of fruit.
- Do 40 sit-ups <u>or</u> hula hoop for 50 seconds in one direction and 50 seconds in the other direction.
- Think of something you like about yourself.
- Eat at least one and a 1/2 cups of vegetables.
- Do something nice for someone else.
- With your arms straight out from your sides, do arm circles 20 forward, 20 backward, big and small.
- Work on achieving your goal(s).
- Hop on one leg and count to 25, then the other and count to 25.
- **Do 3 push-ups (on your knees or on your toes).**

*Health Tip: Yellow fruits and vegetables are good for your skin, teeth, and bones.

Day Sixty-Two

- Drink 6-8 glasses of water (no flavor added, just WATER).
- Go for a walk, jog or march in place for at least 21 minutes.
- Shut off all electronics for 6 minutes. Close your eyes. Inhale slowly and deeply to the count of 4, then exhale slowly to the count of 4.
- Think of something you are thankful for today.
- Stand on one leg and count to 30, stand on the other and count to 30.
- Do 50 Jumping Jacks.
- Eat two whole pieces of fruit.
- Do **45** sit-ups <u>or</u> hula hoop for **55** seconds in one direction and **55** seconds in the other direction.
- Think of something you like about yourself.
- Eat at least one and a 1/2 cups of vegetables.
- Do something nice for someone else.
- With your arms straight out from your sides, do arm circles 20 forward, 20 backward, big and small.
- Work on achieving your goal(s).
- Hop on one leg and count to 25, then the other and count to 25.
- Do 3 push-ups.

*Avoid all electronics today (except for any electronics you need to use for school).

Day Sixty-Three

- Drink 6-8 glasses of water (no flavor added, just WATER).
- Go for a walk, jog or march in place for at least 21 minutes.
- Shut off all electronics for 6 minutes. Close your eyes. Inhale slowly and deeply to the count of 4, then exhale slowly to the count of 4.
- Think of something you are thankful for today.
- Stand on one leg and count to 30, stand on the other and count to 30.
- Do 50 Jumping Jacks.
- Eat two whole pieces of fruit.
- Do 45 sit-ups <u>or</u> hula hoop for 55 seconds in one direction and 55 seconds in the other direction.
- Think of something you like about yourself.
- Eat at least one and a 1/2 cups of vegetables.
- Do something nice for someone else.
- With your arms straight out from your sides, do arm circles 20 forward, 20 backward - **small, medium and large**.
- Work on achieving your goal(s).
- Hop on one leg and count to 25, then the other and count to 25.
- Do 3 push-ups.
- **Decide on a new goal. If you have not completed your first two, keep working on them.**

Day Sixty-Four

- Drink 6-8 glasses of water (no flavor added, just WATER).
- Go for a walk, jog or march in place for at least **23** minutes.
- Shut off all electronics for 6 minutes. Close your eyes. Inhale slowly and deeply to the count of 4, then exhale slowly to the count of 4.
- Think of something you are thankful for today.
- Stand on one leg and count to 30, stand on the other and count to 30.
- Do 50 Jumping Jacks.
- Eat two whole pieces of fruit.
- Do 45 sit-ups or hula hoop for 55 seconds in one direction and 55 seconds in the other direction.
- Think of something you like about yourself.
- Eat at least one and a 1/2 cups of vegetables.
- Do something nice for someone else.
- With your arms straight out from your sides, do arm circles 20 forward, 20 backward - small, medium and large.
- Work on achieving your goal(s).
- Hop on one leg and count to 25, then the other and count to 25.
- Do 3 push-ups.

*Health Tip: Green fruits and vegetables are good for your eyes, bones, and teeth.

Day Sixty-Five

- Drink 6-8 glasses of water (no flavor added, just WATER).
- Go for a walk, jog or march in place for at least **23** minutes.
- Shut off all electronics for 6 minutes. Close your eyes. Inhale slowly and deeply to the count of 4, then exhale slowly to the count of 4.
- Think of something you are thankful for today.
- Stand on one leg and count to 30, stand on the other and count to 30.
- Do 50 Jumping Jacks.
- Eat two whole pieces of fruit.
- Do 45 sit-ups <u>or</u> hula hoop for 55 seconds in one direction and 55 seconds in the other direction.
- Think of something you like about yourself.
- Eat at least one and a 1/2 cups of vegetables.
- Do something nice for someone else.
- With your arms straight out from your sides, do arm circles 20 forward, 20 backward - small, medium and large.
- Work on achieving your goal(s).
- Hop on one leg and count to 25, then the other and count to 25.
- Do 3 push-ups.

*Brain Challenge: Say your ABC's backwards.

Day Sixty-Six

- Drink 6-8 glasses of water (no flavor added, just WATER).
- Go for a walk, jog or march in place for at least 23 minutes.
- Shut off all electronics for 6 minutes. Close your eyes. Inhale slowly and deeply to the count of 4, then exhale slowly to the count of 4.
- Think of something you are thankful for today.
- Stand on one leg and count to 30, stand on the other and count to 30.
- Do **55** Jumping Jacks.
- Eat two whole pieces of fruit.
- Do 45 sit-ups <u>or</u> hula hoop for 55 seconds in one direction and 55 seconds in the other direction.
- Think of something you like about yourself.
- Eat at least one and a 1/2 cups of vegetables.
- Do something nice for someone else.
- With your arms straight out from your sides, do arm circles 20 forward, 20 backward - small, medium and large.
- Work on achieving your goal(s).
- Hop on one leg and count to 25, then the other and count to 25.
- Do 3 push-ups.

*Health Tip: When using electronic devices, it is important to take breaks, look away, and focus on something else for a little while.

Day Sixty-Seven

- Drink 6-8 glasses of water (no flavor added, just WATER).
- Go for a walk, jog or march in place for at least 23 minutes.
- Shut off all electronics for 6 minutes. Close your eyes. Inhale slowly and deeply to the count of 4, then exhale slowly to the count of 4.
- Think of something you are thankful for today.
- Stand on one leg and count to 30, stand on the other and count to 30.
- Do 55 Jumping Jacks.
- Eat two whole pieces of fruit.
- Do 45 sit-ups or hula hoop for 55 seconds in one direction and 55 seconds in the other direction.
- Think of something you like about yourself.
- Eat at least one and a 1/2 cups of vegetables.
- Do something nice for someone else.
- With your arms straight out from your sides, do arm circles 20 forward, 20 backward - small, medium and large.
- Work on achieving your goal(s).
- Hop on one leg and count to 25, then the other and count to 25.
- Do 3 push-ups.

*Just for today, every time you go to your room hop to get there.

Day Sixty-Eight

- Drink 6-8 glasses of water (no flavor added, just WATER).
- Go for a walk, jog or march in place for at least 23 minutes.
- Shut off all electronics for 6 minutes. Close your eyes. Inhale slowly and deeply to the count of 4, then exhale slowly to the count of 4.
- Think of something you are thankful for today.
- Stand on one leg and count to 30, stand on the other and count to 30.
- Do 55 Jumping Jacks.
- Eat two whole pieces of fruit.
- Do 45 sit-ups or hula hoop for 55 seconds in one direction and 55 seconds in the other direction.
- Think of something you like about yourself.
- Eat at least one and a 1/2 cups of vegetables.
- Do something nice for someone else.
- With your arms straight out from your sides, do arm circles 20 forward, 20 backward - small, medium and large.
- Work on achieving your goal(s).
- Hop on one leg and count to 25, then the other and count to 25.
- Do 5 push-ups.

*Health Tip: Studies have found that students who get a good night's sleep tend to get better grades than those who don't.

Day Sixty-Nine

- Drink 6-8 glasses of water (no flavor added, just WATER).
- Go for a walk, jog or march in place for at least 23 minutes.
- Shut off all electronics for 6 minutes. Close your eyes. Inhale slowly and deeply to the count of 4, then exhale slowly to the count of 4.
- Think of something you are thankful for today.
- Stand on one leg and count to 30, stand on the other and count to 30.
- Do 55 Jumping Jacks.
- Eat two whole pieces of fruit.
- Do **50** sit-ups <u>or</u> hula hoop for **60** seconds in one direction and **60** seconds in the other direction.
- Think of something you like about yourself.
- Eat at least one and a 1/2 cups of vegetables.
- Do something nice for someone else.
- With your arms straight out from your sides, do arm circles 20 forward, 20 backward - small, medium and large.
- Work on achieving your goal(s).
- Hop on one leg and count to 25, then the other and count to 25.
- Do 5 push-ups.

*Health Tip: Tomatoes and strawberries are good for your heart.

Day Seventy

- Drink 6-8 glasses of water (no flavor added, just WATER).
- Go for a walk, jog or march in place for at least 23 minutes.
- Shut off all electronics for 6 minutes. Close your eyes. Inhale slowly and deeply to the count of 4, then exhale slowly to the count of 4.
- Think of something you are thankful for today.
- Stand on one leg and count to 30, stand on the other and count to 30.
- Do 55 Jumping Jacks.
- Eat two whole pieces of fruit.
- Do 50 sit-ups or hula hoop for 60 seconds in one direction and 60 seconds in the other direction.
- Think of something you like about yourself.
- Eat at least one and a 1/2 cups of vegetables.
- Do something nice for someone else.
- With your arms straight out from your sides, do arm circles **25** forward, **25** backward - small, medium and large.
- Work on achieving your goal(s).
- Hop on one leg and count to 25, then the other and count to 25.
- Do 5 push-ups.

*Health Tip: Avoid watching commercials, they are designed to make you crave the unhealthy foods that the company is trying to sell.

Day Seventy-One

- Drink 6-8 glasses of water (no flavor added, just WATER).
- Go for a walk, jog or march in place for at least **25** minutes.
- Shut off all electronics for 6 minutes. Close your eyes. Inhale slowly and deeply to the count of 4, then exhale slowly to the count of 4.
- Think of something you are thankful for today.
- Stand on one leg and count to 30, stand on the other and count to 30.
- Do 55 Jumping Jacks.
- Eat two whole pieces of fruit.
- Do 50 sit-ups <u>or</u> hula hoop for 60 seconds in one direction and 60 seconds in the other direction.
- Think of something you like about yourself.
- Eat at least one and a 1/2 cups of vegetables.
- Do something nice for someone else.
- With your arms straight out from your sides, do arm circles 25 forward, 25 backward - small, medium and large.
- Work on achieving your goal(s).
- Hop on one leg and count to 25, then the other and count to 25.
- Do 5 push-ups.

*Health Tip: Staying well hydrated keeps your skin and lips from drying out. It also helps you keep cool during the summer.

Day Seventy-Two

- Drink 6-8 glasses of water (no flavor added, just WATER).
- Go for a walk, jog or march in place for at least 25 minutes.
- Shut off all electronics for 6 minutes. Close your eyes. Inhale slowly and deeply to the count of 4, then exhale slowly to the count of 4.
- Think of something you are thankful for today.
- Stand on one leg and count to **35**, stand on the other and count to **30**.
- Do 55 Jumping Jacks.
- Eat two whole pieces of fruit.
- Do 50 sit-ups or hula hoop for 60 seconds in one direction and 60 seconds in the other direction.
- Think of something you like about yourself.
- Eat at least one and a 1/2 cups of vegetables.
- Do something nice for someone else.
- With your arms straight out from your sides, do arm circles 25 forward, 25 backward - small, medium and large.
- Work on achieving your goal(s).
- Hop on one leg and count to 25, then the other and count to 25.
- Do 5 push-ups.

*Just for today, every time you go to your kitchen, skip to get there.

Day Seventy-Three

- Drink 6-8 glasses of water (no flavor added, just WATER).
- Go for a walk, jog or march in place for at least 25 minutes.
- Shut off all electronics for 6 minutes. Close your eyes. Inhale slowly and deeply to the count of 4, then exhale slowly to the count of 4.
- Think of something you are thankful for today.
- Stand on one leg and count to 35, stand on the other and count to 30.
- Do **60** Jumping Jacks.
- Eat two whole pieces of fruit.
- Do 50 sit-ups <u>or</u> hula hoop for 60 seconds in one direction and 60 seconds in the other direction.
- Think of something you like about yourself.
- Eat at least one and a 1/2 cups of vegetables.
- Do something nice for someone else.
- With your arms straight out from your sides, do arm circles 25 forward, 25 backward - small, medium and large.
- Work on achieving your goal(s).
- Hop on one leg and count to 25, then the other and count to 25.
- Do 5 push-ups.

*Health Tip: Sweet potatoes are good for your eyes and your immunity.

Day Seventy-Four

- Drink 6-8 glasses of water (no flavor added, just WATER).
- Go for a walk, jog or march in place for at least 25 minutes.
- Shut off all electronics for 6 minutes. Close your eyes. Inhale slowly and deeply to the count of 4, then exhale slowly to the count of 4.
- Think of something you are thankful for today.
- Stand on one leg and count to 35, stand on the other and count to 30.
- Do 60 Jumping Jacks.
- Eat two whole pieces of fruit.
- Do 50 sit-ups or hula hoop for 60 seconds in one direction and 60 seconds in the other direction.
- Think of something you like about yourself.
- Eat at least one and a 1/2 cups of vegetables.
- Do something nice for someone else.
- With your arms straight out from your sides, do arm circles 25 forward, 25 backward - small, medium and large.
- Work on achieving your goal(s).
- Hop on one leg and count to 25, then the other and count to 25.
- Do 5 push-ups.

*Health Tip: Just 5 minutes of anger can impair your immune system for 6 hours. Forgive others and be happy for your health.

Day Seventy-Five

- Drink 6-8 glasses of water (no flavor added, just WATER).
- Go for a walk, jog or march in place for at least 25 minutes.
- Shut off all electronics for 6 minutes. Close your eyes. Inhale slowly and deeply to the count of 4, then exhale slowly to the count of 4.
- Think of something you are thankful for today.
- Stand on one leg and count to 35, stand on the other and count to 30.
- Do 60 Jumping Jacks.
- Eat two whole pieces of fruit.
- Do 50 sit-ups or hula hoop for 60 seconds in one direction and 60 seconds in the other direction.
- Think of something you like about yourself.
- Eat at least one and a 1/2 cups of vegetables.
- Do something nice for someone else.
- With your arms straight out from your sides, do arm circles 25 forward, 25 backward - small, medium and large.
- Work on achieving your goal(s).
- Hop on one leg and count to 25, then the other and count to 25.
- Do 7 push-ups.

*Brain Challenge: Brush your teeth with your left hand (if you are right handed), if you are left handed - use your right hand.

Day Seventy-Six

- Drink 6-8 glasses of water (no flavor added, just WATER).
- Go for a walk, jog or march in place for at least 25 minutes.
- Shut off all electronics for 6 minutes. Close your eyes. Inhale slowly and deeply to the count of 4, then exhale slowly to the count of 4.
- Think of something you are thankful for today.
- Stand on one leg and count to 35, stand on the other and count to 30.
- Do 60 Jumping Jacks.
- Eat two whole pieces of fruit.
- Do 50 sit-ups or hula hoop for 60 seconds in one direction and 60 seconds in the other direction.
- Think of something you like about yourself.
- Eat at least one and a 1/2 cups of vegetables.
- Do something nice for someone else.
- With your arms straight out from your sides, do arm circles 25 forward, 25 backward - small, medium and large.
- Work on achieving your goal(s).
- Hop on one leg and count to 25, then the other and count to 25.
- Do 7 push-ups.

*Health Tip: Choosing whole grain bread and brown rice over white bread and white rice is good for your heart and your digestion (your body's process to break down food).

Day Seventy-Seven

- Drink 6-8 glasses of water (no flavor added, just WATER).
- Go for a walk, jog or march in place for at least 25 minutes.
- Shut off all electronics for 6 minutes. Close your eyes. Inhale slowly and deeply to the count of 4, then exhale slowly to the count of 4.
- Think of something you are thankful for today.
- Stand on one leg and count to 35, stand on the other and count to 30.
- Do 60 Jumping Jacks.
- Eat two whole pieces of fruit.
- Do 50 sit-ups or hula hoop for 60 seconds in one direction and 60 seconds in the other direction.
- Think of something you like about yourself.
- Eat at least one and a 1/2 cups of vegetables.
- Do something nice for someone else.
- With your arms straight out from your sides, do arm circles **30** forward, **30** backward - small, medium and large.
- Work on achieving your goal(s).
- Hop on one leg and count to **30**, then the other and count to **30**.
- Do 7 push-ups.

*Health Tip: Dancing is a great way to exercise because it's fun, boosts your mood, and is good for your heart and lungs.

Day Seventy-Eight

- Drink 6-8 glasses of water (no flavor added, just WATER).
- Go for a walk, jog or march in place for at least **27** minutes.
- Shut off all electronics for 6 minutes. Close your eyes. Inhale slowly and deeply to the count of 4, then exhale slowly to the count of 4.
- Think of something you are thankful for today.
- Stand on one leg and count to 35, stand on the other and count to 30.
- Do 60 Jumping Jacks.
- Eat two whole pieces of fruit.
- Do 50 sit-ups or hula hoop for 60 seconds in one direction and 60 seconds in the other direction.
- Think of something you like about yourself.
- Eat at least one and a 1/2 cups of vegetables.
- Do something nice for someone else.
- With your arms straight out from your sides, do arm circles 30 forward, 30 backward - small, medium and large.
- Work on achieving your goal(s).
- Hop on one leg and count to 30, then the other and count to 30.
- Do 7 push-ups.

*Just for today, every time you sit down (while you are at home), stand up and sit down again 3x.

Day Seventy-Nine

- Drink 6-8 glasses of water (no flavor added, just WATER).
- Go for a walk, jog or march in place for at least 27 minutes.
- Shut off all electronics for 6 minutes. Close your eyes. Inhale slowly and deeply to the count of 4, then exhale slowly to the count of 4.
- Think of something you are thankful for today.
- Stand on one leg and count to **40**, stand on the other and count to **40**.
- Do 60 Jumping Jacks.
- Eat two whole pieces of fruit.
- Do 50 sit-ups <u>or</u> hula hoop for 60 seconds in one direction and 60 seconds in the other direction.
- Think of something you like about yourself.
- Eat at least one and a 1/2 cups of vegetables.
- Do something nice for someone else.
- With your arms straight out from your sides, do arm circles 30 forward, 30 backward - small, medium and large.
- Work on achieving your goal(s).
- Hop on one leg and count to 30, then the other and count to 30.
- Do 7 push-ups.

*Health Tip: The caffeine in coffee and soda isn't good for you. It can increase your heart rate and blood pressure; make you feel anxious; and make it hard to sleep.

Day Eighty

- Drink 6-8 glasses of water (no flavor added, just WATER).
- Go for a walk, jog or march in place for at least 27 minutes.
- Shut off all electronics for 6 minutes. Close your eyes. Inhale slowly and deeply to the count of 4, then exhale slowly to the count of 4.
- Think of something you are thankful for today.
- Stand on one leg and count to 40, stand on the other and count to 40.
- Do 60 Jumping Jacks.
- Eat two whole pieces of fruit.
- Do 50 sit-ups <u>or</u> hula hoop for 60 seconds in one direction and 60 seconds in the other direction.
- Think of something you like about yourself.
- Eat at least one and a 1/2 cups of vegetables.
- Do something nice for someone else.
- With your arms straight out from your sides, do arm circles 30 forward, 30 backward - small, medium and large.
- Work on achieving your goal(s).
- Hop on one leg and count to 30, then the other and count to 30.
- Do 7 push-ups.

*Health Tip: Swimming is good for your heart and your lungs.

Day Eighty-One

- Drink 6-8 glasses of water (no flavor added, just WATER).
- Go for a walk, jog or march in place for at least 27 minutes.
- Shut off all electronics for 6 minutes. Close your eyes. Inhale slowly and deeply to the count of 4, then exhale slowly to the count of 4.
- Think of something you are thankful for today.
- Stand on one leg and count to 40, stand on the other and count to 40.
- Do 60 Jumping Jacks.
- Eat two whole pieces of fruit.
- Do 50 sit-ups or hula hoop for 60 seconds in one direction and 60 seconds in the other direction.
- Think of something you like about yourself.
- Eat at least one and a 1/2 cups of vegetables.
- Do something nice for someone else.
- With your arms straight out from your sides, do arm circles 30 forward, 30 backward - small, medium and large.
- Work on achieving your goal(s).
- Hop on one leg and count to 30, then the other and count to 30.
- Do 7 push-ups.

*Avoid all electronics today (except for any electronics you need to use for school).

Day Eighty-Two

- Drink 6-8 glasses of water (no flavor added, just WATER).
- Go for a walk, jog or march in place for at least 27 minutes.
- Shut off all electronics for 6 minutes. Close your eyes. Inhale slowly and deeply to the count of 4, then exhale slowly to the count of 4.
- Think of something you are thankful for today.
- Stand on one leg and count to 40, stand on the other and count to 40.
- Do 60 Jumping Jacks.
- Eat two whole pieces of fruit.
- Do 50 sit-ups or hula hoop for 60 seconds in one direction and 60 seconds in the other direction.
- Think of something you like about yourself.
- Eat at least one and a 1/2 cups of vegetables.
- Do something nice for someone else.
- With your arms straight out from your sides, do arm circles 30 forward, 30 backward - small, medium and large.
- Work on achieving your goal(s).
- Hop on one leg and count to 30, then the other and count to 30.
- Do 9 push-ups.

*Relaxation Technique: Tense yourself all over (feet, hands, legs, arms, shoulders, and stomach) for four or five seconds. Then let go all at once.

Day Eighty-Three

- Drink 6-8 glasses of water (no flavor added, just WATER).
- Go for a walk, jog or march in place for at least 27 minutes.
- Shut off all electronics for 6 minutes. Close your eyes. Inhale slowly and deeply to the count of 4, then exhale slowly to the count of 4.
- Think of something you are thankful for today.
- Stand on one leg and count to 40, stand on the other and count to 40.
- Do 60 Jumping Jacks.
- Eat two whole pieces of fruit.
- Do 50 sit-ups <u>or</u> hula hoop for 60 seconds in one direction and 60 seconds in the other direction.
- Think of something you like about yourself.
- Eat at least one and a 1/2 cups of vegetables.
- Do something nice for someone else.
- With your arms straight out from your sides, do arm circles 30 forward, 30 backward - small, medium and large.
- Work on achieving your goal(s).
- Hop on one leg and count to 30, then the other and count to 30.
- Do 9 push-ups.

*Health Tip: Blueberries are good for your brain, heart, and skin.

Day Eighty-Four

- Drink 6-8 glasses of water (no flavor added, just WATER).
- Go for a walk, jog or march in place for at least 27 minutes.
- Shut off all electronics for 6 minutes. Close your eyes. Inhale slowly and deeply to the count of 4, then exhale slowly to the count of 4.
- Think of something you are thankful for today.
- Stand on one leg and count to 40, stand on the other and count to 40.
- Do 60 Jumping Jacks.
- Eat two whole pieces of fruit.
- Do 50 sit-ups or hula hoop for 60 seconds in one direction and 60 seconds in the other direction.
- Think of something you like about yourself.
- Eat at least one and a 1/2 cups of vegetables.
- Do something nice for someone else.
- With your arms straight out from your sides, do arm circles 30 forward, 30 backward - small, medium and large.
- Work on achieving your goal(s).
- Hop on one leg and count to 30, then the other and count to 30.
- Do 9 push-ups.

*Health Tip: Riding your bike is a great exercise because it strengthens your legs and improves balance.

Day Eighty-Five

- Drink 6-8 glasses of water (no flavor added, just WATER).
- Go for a walk, jog or march in place for at least 27 minutes.
- Shut off all electronics for 6 minutes. Close your eyes. Inhale slowly and deeply to the count of 4, then exhale slowly to the count of 4.
- Think of something you are thankful for today.
- Stand on one leg and count to 40, stand on the other and count to 40.
- Do 60 Jumping Jacks.
- Eat two whole pieces of fruit.
- Do 50 sit-ups or hula hoop for 60 seconds in one direction and 60 seconds in the other direction.
- Think of something you like about yourself.
- Eat at least one and a 1/2 cups of vegetables.
- Do something nice for someone else.
- With your arms straight out from your sides, do arm circles 30 forward, 30 backward - small, medium and large.
- Work on achieving your goal(s).
- Hop on one leg and count to 30, then the other and count to 30.
- Do 9 push-ups.

*Brain Challenge: Use your left hand when you eat dinner tonight (if you are right handed), if you are left handed use your right hand.

Day Eighty-Six

- Drink 6-8 glasses of water (no flavor added, just WATER).
- Go for a walk, jog or march in place for at least 27 minutes.
- Shut off all electronics for 6 minutes. Close your eyes. Inhale slowly and deeply to the count of 4, then exhale slowly to the count of 4.
- Think of something you are thankful for today.
- Stand on one leg and count to **45**, stand on the other and count to **45**.
- Do 60 Jumping Jacks.
- Eat two whole pieces of fruit.
- Do 50 sit-ups or hula hoop for 60 seconds in one direction and 60 seconds in the other direction.
- Think of something you like about yourself.
- Eat at least one and a 1/2 cups of vegetables.
- Do something nice for someone else.
- With your arms straight out from your sides, do arm circles 30 forward, 30 backward - small, medium and large.
- Work on achieving your goal(s).
- Hop on one leg and count to **40**, then the other and count to **40**.
- Do 9 push-ups.

*Health Tip: Spinach strengthens your bones and keeps your hair and skin healthy.

Day Eighty-Seven

- Drink 6-8 glasses of water (no flavor added, just WATER).
- Go for a walk, jog or march in place for at least 27 minutes.
- Shut off all electronics for 6 minutes. Close your eyes. Inhale slowly and deeply to the count of 4, then exhale slowly to the count of 4.
- Think of something you are thankful for today.
- Stand on one leg and count to 45, stand on the other and count to 45.
- Do 60 Jumping Jacks.
- Eat two whole pieces of fruit.
- Do 50 sit-ups or hula hoop for 60 seconds in one direction and 60 seconds in the other direction.
- Think of something you like about yourself.
- Eat at least one and a 1/2 cups of vegetables.
- Do something nice for someone else.
- With your arms straight out from your sides, do arm circles 30 forward, 30 backward - small, medium and large.
- Work on achieving your goal(s).
- Hop on one leg and count to 40, then the other and count to 40.
- Do 9 push-ups.

*Test Yourself: How many sit-ups can you do in 2 minutes?

Day Eighty-Eight

- Drink 6-8 glasses of water (no flavor added, just WATER).
- Go for a walk, jog or march in place for at least 27 minutes.
- Shut off all electronics for 6 minutes. Close your eyes. Inhale slowly and deeply to the count of 4, then exhale slowly to the count of 4.
- Think of something you are thankful for today.
- Stand on one leg and count to 45, stand on the other and count to 45.
- Do 60 Jumping Jacks.
- Eat two whole pieces of fruit.
- Do 50 sit-ups or hula hoop for 60 seconds in one direction and 60 seconds in the other direction.
- Think of something you like about yourself.
- Eat at least one and a 1/2 cups of vegetables.
- Do something nice for someone else.
- With your arms straight out from your sides, do arm circles 30 forward, 30 backward - small, medium and large.
- Work on achieving your goal(s).
- Hop on one leg and count to 40, then the other and count to 40.
- Do 9 push-ups.

*Test Yourself: How many jumping jacks can you do in 2 minutes?

Day Eighty-Nine

- Drink 6-8 glasses of water (no flavor added, just WATER).
- Go for a walk, jog or march in place for at least 27 minutes.
- Shut off all electronics for 6 minutes. Close your eyes. Inhale slowly and deeply to the count of 4, then exhale slowly to the count of 4.
- Think of something you are thankful for today.
- Stand on one leg and count to 45, stand on the other and count to 45.
- Do 60 Jumping Jacks.
- Eat two whole pieces of fruit.
- Do 50 sit-ups <u>or</u> hula hoop for 60 seconds in one direction and 60 seconds in the other direction.
- Think of something you like about yourself.
- Eat at least one and a 1/2 cups of vegetables.
- Do something nice for someone else.
- With your arms straight out from your sides, do arm circles 30 forward, 30 backward - small, medium and large.
- Work on achieving your goal(s).
- Hop on one leg and count to 40, then the other and count to 40.
- Do **10** push-ups.

*Test Yourself: How long can you sit quietly, while closing your eyes and inhaling and exhaling slowly.

Day Ninety

- Drink 6-8 glasses of water (no flavor added, just WATER).
- Go for a walk, jog or march in place for at least 27 minutes.
- Shut off all electronics for 6 minutes. Close your eyes. Inhale slowly and deeply to the count of 4, then exhale slowly to the count of 4.
- Think of something you are thankful for today.
- Stand on one leg and count to 45, stand on the other and count to 45.
- Do 60 Jumping Jacks.
- Eat two whole pieces of fruit.
- Do 50 sit-ups <u>or</u> hula hoop for 60 seconds in one direction and 60 seconds in the other direction.
- Think of something you like about yourself.
- Eat at least one and a 1/2 cups of vegetables.
- Do something nice for someone else.
- With your arms straight out from your sides, do arm circles 30 forward, 30 backward - small, medium and large.
- Work on achieving your goal(s).
- Hop on one leg and count to 40, then the other and count to 40.
- Do 10 push-ups.

*Don't stop now, keep going!

Every Day From Now On

For optimal function of every organ in your body:
- Drink **at least** 6-8 glasses of water (no flavor added, just WATER).

To maintain a healthy body and mind, and to prevent diseases:
- Go for a walk or jog, or march in place or try another activity such as swimming or biking for **at least** 30 minutes.
- Shut off all electronics for **at least** 6 minutes. Close your eyes. Inhale slowly and deeply to the count of 4, then exhale slowly to the count of 4 (breathe this way until time is up).
- Hop on one leg and count to **at least** 40, then the other and count to **at least** 40.
- Do **at least** 60 Jumping Jacks.
- Do **at least** 50 sit-ups or hula hoop for **at least** 60 seconds in both directions.
- Do **at least** 30 arm circles forward, and **at least** 30 backward, small, medium, and large.
- Do **at least** 10 push-ups.
- Eat **at least** two whole pieces of fruit.
- Eat **at least** one and a half cups of vegetables.

To stay confident, positive, and happy:
- Continue to work on your goals and create new ones.
- Think of something you are thankful for.
- Think of something you like about yourself.
- Do something nice for someone else.